APPENDIX CANCER COOKBOOK

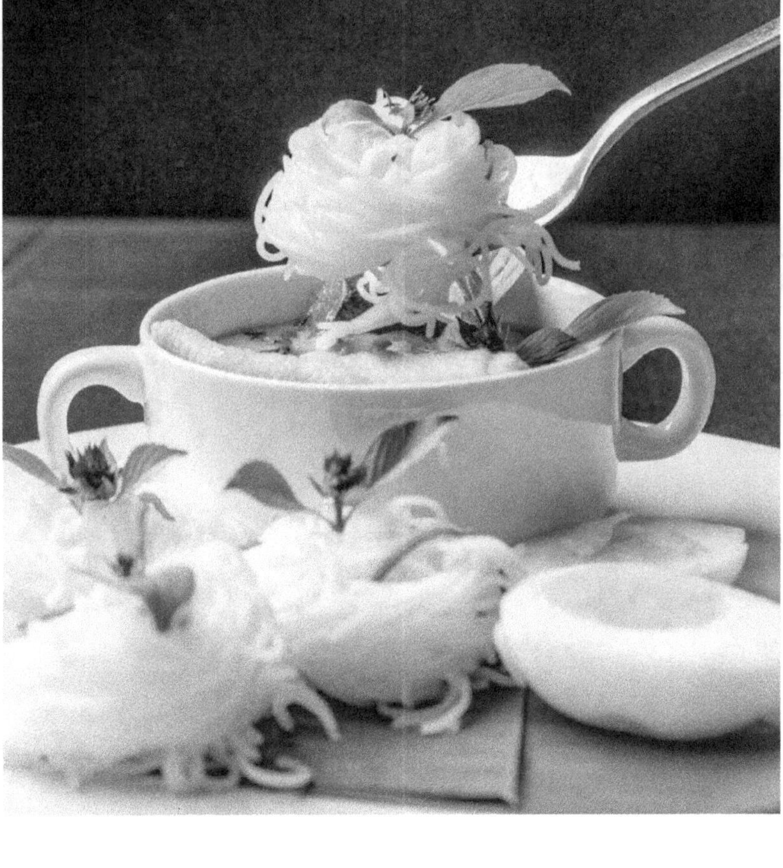

This book belongs to...

Appendix Cancer Cookbook

Recipes to Nourish and Boost Health

-- Drusilla Ronnell Allison --

Attribution

This cover was designed with help from pexels.com

ISBN

9798321216668

Imprint

Independently Published

== Disclaimer ==

The information contained in this book is for general informational purposes only. The author and publisher have made every effort to ensure that the content provided is accurate and up-to-date at the time of publication. However, medical knowledge is constantly evolving, and individual circumstances vary. Therefore, the author and publisher do not make any representations or warranties of any kind, express or implied, about the completeness, accuracy, reliability, suitability, or availability of the information contained in this book.

The information provided is not a substitute for professional medical advice, diagnosis, or treatment. Always seek the advice of your physician or another qualified healthcare provider with any questions you may have regarding a medical condition. Never disregard professional medical advice or delay seeking it because of something you have read in this book.

The author and publisher disclaim any responsibility for any adverse effects resulting directly or indirectly from the use of the information provided in this book. The reader assumes full responsibility for consulting a qualified healthcare professional regarding health conditions and before starting any new treatment or making changes to existing treatment.

The inclusion of specific products, services, or medical procedures in this book does not imply endorsement. The author and publisher shall have no liability for any damages or loss arising out of, or in connection with, the use of this book.

It is recommended to independently verify any information provided in this book and consult with a qualified healthcare professional for advice tailored to your individual circumstances.

List of Contents

Personal Note for This Cookbook

As you embark on the journey through these pages, I want to extend my heartfelt support and encouragement. This cookbook is not just a collection of recipes; it's a reflection of the love and care that goes into nourishing oneself and others during challenging times.

I hope these recipes bring comfort, joy, and strength to your table, reminding you that nourishing your body is an act of self-love and resilience. Remember, you are not alone in this journey, and together, we can find solace and sustenance in the simple pleasure of sharing a meal.

Important note about this book: Please note that the information provided here is for general knowledge and should not replace professional medical advice. If you have specific concerns or questions about **Appendix Cancer**, it's best to consult with a healthcare professional familiar with your medical history.

1. Introduction

Welcome to the "Appendix Cancer Cookbook." This cookbook is crafted with care and compassion to provide a collection of nourishing and flavorful recipes tailored specifically for individuals navigating through the challenges of appendix cancer treatment and recovery.

Living with cancer brings forth a unique set of dietary considerations. During treatment, maintaining proper nutrition is essential to support the body's strength and resilience, while also managing potential side effects such as nausea, fatigue, and loss of appetite. As patients progress through their journey, wholesome meals play a crucial role in promoting healing, restoring energy, and enhancing overall well-being.

In this cookbook, you'll find a diverse range of recipes thoughtfully curated to meet the nutritional needs of appendix cancer patients and survivors. From comforting soups and hearty salads to satisfying main courses and nutritious snacks, each recipe is designed to nourish the body and delight the palate.

Drawing inspiration from various cuisines and incorporating nutrient-rich ingredients, these recipes prioritize flavor, texture, and ease of preparation. Whether you're seeking light and refreshing dishes or hearty and comforting meals, you'll discover a wealth of options to suit your taste preferences and dietary requirements.

We understand that maintaining a balanced diet can be challenging amidst the demands of cancer treatment. That's why each recipe in this cookbook is crafted with simplicity in mind, utilizing accessible ingredients and straightforward cooking techniques. Whether you're cooking for yourself or preparing meals for loved ones, these recipes aim to simplify mealtime while providing delicious and wholesome options.

As you embark on your culinary journey through this cookbook, we hope these recipes inspire creativity, nourish the body, and bring joy to your kitchen. May each meal serve as a source of comfort, strength, and vitality as you navigate through your appendix cancer journey.

Here's to nourishment, resilience, and the healing power of food.

2. Healing Vegetable Soup

Ingredients:

- 2 carrots, diced

- 2 celery stalks, diced

- 1 onion, diced

- 2 cloves garlic, minced

- 1 tablespoon olive oil

- 6 cups low-sodium vegetable broth

- 1 cup diced tomatoes

- 1 cup chopped spinach or kale

- 1 teaspoon turmeric powder

- Salt and pepper to taste

- Fresh herbs like parsley or cilantro for garnish

Instructions:

1. In a large pot, heat olive oil over medium heat. Add onions, carrots, celery, and garlic. Sauté until onions are translucent.

2. Pour in the vegetable broth and bring to a simmer.

3. Add diced tomatoes, turmeric powder, salt, and pepper. Let the soup simmer for 20-25 minutes.

4. Stir in chopped spinach or kale and cook for an additional 5 minutes.

5. Adjust seasoning if necessary. Serve hot, garnished with fresh herbs.

3. Quinoa and Chickpea Salad

Ingredients:

- 1 cup quinoa, rinsed
- 1 can chickpeas, drained and rinsed
- 1 cucumber, diced
- 1 bell pepper, diced
- 1/4 cup chopped fresh parsley
- 1/4 cup chopped fresh mint
- Juice of 1 lemon
- 2 tablespoons olive oil
- Salt and pepper to taste

Instructions:

1. Cook quinoa according to package instructions. Let it cool.

2. In a large bowl, combine cooked quinoa, chickpeas, cucumber, bell pepper, parsley, and mint.

3. In a small bowl, whisk together lemon juice, olive oil, salt, and pepper.

4. Pour the dressing over the salad and toss until everything is well coated.

5. Refrigerate for at least 30 minutes before serving to allow flavors to meld.

4. Baked Salmon with Lemon and Dill

Ingredients:

- 4 salmon fillets

- 2 tablespoons olive oil

- Juice of 1 lemon

- 2 cloves garlic, minced

- 2 tablespoons chopped fresh dill

- Salt and pepper to taste

- Lemon slices for garnish

Instructions:

1. Preheat the oven to 375°F (190°C).

2. In a small bowl, whisk together olive oil, lemon juice, minced garlic, chopped dill, salt, and pepper.

3. Place salmon fillets on a baking sheet lined with parchment paper.

4. Brush the salmon fillets with the prepared marinade, coating them evenly.

5. Place lemon slices on top of each fillet.

6. Bake in the preheated oven for 12-15 minutes, or until the salmon is cooked through and flakes easily with a fork.

7. Serve hot, garnished with additional fresh dill if desired.

5. Immune-Boosting Green Smoothie

Ingredients:

- 1 cup spinach
- 1/2 cup kale
- 1 small ripe banana
- 1/2 cup frozen mixed berries
- 1/2 cup unsweetened almond milk (or any milk of your choice)
- 1 tablespoon honey or maple syrup (optional)
- 1/2 inch piece of fresh ginger, peeled and grated (optional)
- 1 tablespoon chia seeds (optional)

Instructions:

1. Place all ingredients in a blender.
2. Blend until smooth and creamy, adding more almond milk if needed to reach your desired consistency.
3. Taste and adjust sweetness if necessary by adding honey or maple syrup.
4. Pour into glasses and serve immediately for maximum freshness and nutrients.

6. Turmeric-Ginger Tea

Ingredients:

- 2 cups water

- 1 teaspoon ground turmeric

- 1/2 teaspoon ground ginger (or 1-inch piece of fresh ginger, sliced)

- 1 tablespoon honey (optional)

- Juice of 1/2 lemon (optional)

Instructions:

1. In a small saucepan, bring water to a boil.

2. Add turmeric and ginger to the boiling water.

3. Reduce heat to low and let the mixture simmer for 10 minutes.

4. Strain the tea into cups.

5. Stir in honey and lemon juice if desired.

6. Enjoy this comforting and immune-boosting beverage.

7. Oatmeal Breakfast Bowl

Ingredients:

- 1/2 cup rolled oats

- 1 cup almond milk (or any milk of your choice)

- 1 tablespoon chia seeds

- 1/2 teaspoon ground cinnamon

- 1 ripe banana, sliced

- 1 tablespoon almond butter (or peanut butter)

- Fresh berries for topping

Instructions:

1. In a small saucepan, combine rolled oats and almond milk.

2. Bring to a simmer over medium heat, stirring occasionally.

3. Once the oats start to thicken, stir in chia seeds and ground cinnamon.

4. Cook for another 2-3 minutes until the oats are creamy and fully cooked.

5. Transfer the oatmeal to a bowl and top with sliced banana, almond butter, and fresh berries.

6. Enjoy a hearty and nutritious breakfast that will keep you energized throughout the day.

8. Roasted Vegetable Medley

Ingredients:

- 2 cups mixed vegetables (such as carrots, bell peppers, zucchini, and broccoli), chopped into bite-sized pieces

- 2 tablespoons olive oil

- 2 cloves garlic, minced

- 1 teaspoon dried herbs (such as thyme, rosemary, or oregano)

- Salt and pepper to taste

Instructions:

1. Preheat the oven to 400°F (200°C).

2. In a large bowl, toss the mixed vegetables with olive oil, minced garlic, dried herbs, salt, and pepper until evenly coated.

3. Spread the vegetables in a single layer on a baking sheet lined with parchment paper.

4. Roast in the preheated oven for 20-25 minutes, or until the vegetables are tender and slightly caramelized, stirring halfway through.

5. Serve as a side dish or add to salads and grain bowls for a nutritious boost.

9. Protein-Packed Lentil Soup

Ingredients:

- 1 cup dried lentils, rinsed
- 4 cups vegetable broth
- 1 onion, diced
- 2 carrots, diced
- 2 celery stalks, diced
- 2 cloves garlic, minced
- 1 can diced tomatoes
- 1 teaspoon ground cumin
- 1 teaspoon paprika
- Salt and pepper to taste
- Fresh parsley for garnish

Instructions:

1. In a large pot, combine lentils, vegetable broth, diced tomatoes (with their juices), onion, carrots, celery, garlic, cumin, paprika, salt, and pepper.

2. Bring the mixture to a boil, then reduce heat and let it simmer for 25-30 minutes, or until the lentils and vegetables are tender.

3. Taste and adjust seasoning if needed.

4. Serve hot, garnished with fresh parsley.

10.Greek Yogurt Parfait

Ingredients:

- 1 cup Greek yogurt

- 1/2 cup mixed berries (such as strawberries, blueberries, and raspberries)

- 1/4 cup granola

- 1 tablespoon honey (optional)

Instructions:

1. In a serving glass or bowl, layer Greek yogurt, mixed berries, and granola.

2. Drizzle honey on top if desired for added sweetness.

3. Repeat layers if making multiple servings.

4. Enjoy this delicious and protein-rich parfait as a snack or dessert.

11.Avocado Toast with Poached Egg

Ingredients:

- 2 slices whole grain bread

- 1 ripe avocado

- 2 eggs

- Salt and pepper to taste

- Red pepper flakes (optional)

- Chopped fresh herbs such as parsley or chives (optional)

Instructions:

1. Toast the slices of whole grain bread until golden brown.

2. While the bread is toasting, mash the ripe avocado in a bowl and season with salt and pepper.

3. Poach the eggs to your desired level of doneness.

   - To poach eggs, bring a pot of water to a gentle simmer, then carefully crack the eggs into the water and cook for about 3-4 minutes until the whites are set but the yolks are still runny.

4. Spread the mashed avocado evenly on the toasted bread slices.

5. Carefully place a poached egg on top of each avocado toast.

6. Season with additional salt, pepper, and red pepper flakes if desired.

7. Garnish with chopped fresh herbs for added flavor.

8. Serve immediately for a satisfying and nutritious meal.

12. Spinach and Feta Stuffed Chicken Breast

Ingredients:

- 2 boneless, skinless chicken breasts
- 2 cups fresh spinach leaves
- 1/2 cup crumbled feta cheese
- 2 cloves garlic, minced
- Salt and pepper to taste
- Olive oil for cooking

Instructions:

1. Preheat the oven to 375°F (190°C).

2. Butterfly each chicken breast by slicing horizontally through the thickest part, but not all the way through, to create a pocket.

3. In a bowl, mix together spinach, feta cheese, minced garlic, salt, and pepper.

4. Stuff each chicken breast with the spinach and feta mixture, then secure with toothpicks if needed.

5. Heat olive oil in an oven-safe skillet over medium-high heat.

6. Sear the stuffed chicken breasts for 2-3 minutes on each side until golden brown.

7. Transfer the skillet to the preheated oven and bake for 20-25 minutes, or until the chicken is cooked through and no longer pink in the center.

8. Remove the toothpicks before serving.

9. Slice the stuffed chicken breasts and serve with your favorite side dishes for a wholesome meal.

13.Berry Blast Smoothie Bowl

Ingredients:

- 1 frozen banana

- 1/2 cup mixed berries (such as strawberries, blueberries, and raspberries)

- 1/2 cup unsweetened almond milk (or any milk of your choice)

- 1 tablespoon chia seeds

- Toppings: sliced fresh fruit, granola, shredded coconut, nuts, seeds, or honey (optional)

Instructions:

1. In a blender, combine frozen banana, mixed berries, almond milk, and chia seeds.

2. Blend until smooth and creamy, adding more almond milk if needed to reach your desired consistency.

3. Pour the smoothie into a bowl.

4. Top with sliced fresh fruit, granola, shredded coconut, nuts, seeds, or a drizzle of honey if desired.

5. Enjoy this refreshing and nutritious smoothie bowl for breakfast or as a satisfying snack.

14. Sweet Potato and Black Bean Tacos

Ingredients:

- 2 large sweet potatoes, peeled and diced

- 1 can black beans, drained and rinsed

- 1 teaspoon chili powder

- 1/2 teaspoon ground cumin

- 1/2 teaspoon paprika

- Salt and pepper to taste

- 8 small tortillas (corn or flour)

- Toppings: diced avocado, shredded lettuce, chopped tomatoes, salsa, Greek yogurt or sour cream, lime wedges

Instructions:

1. Preheat the oven to 400°F (200°C).

2. Place diced sweet potatoes on a baking sheet lined with parchment paper. Drizzle with olive oil and sprinkle with chili powder, cumin, paprika, salt, and pepper. Toss to coat evenly.

3. Roast sweet potatoes in the preheated oven for 20-25 minutes, or until tender and slightly caramelized, stirring halfway through.

4. In a small saucepan, heat black beans over medium heat. Stir in a pinch of chili powder, cumin, and salt. Cook until heated through.

5. Warm tortillas in a dry skillet or microwave.

6. Assemble tacos by filling each tortilla with roasted sweet potatoes and black beans. Top with diced avocado, shredded lettuce, chopped tomatoes, salsa, Greek yogurt or sour cream, and a squeeze of lime juice.

7. Serve immediately and enjoy these flavorful and satisfying tacos.

15.Coconut Curry Lentil Soup

Ingredients:

- 1 cup dried red lentils, rinsed

- 1 can coconut milk

- 4 cups vegetable broth

- 1 onion, diced

- 2 cloves garlic, minced

- 1 tablespoon curry powder

- 1 teaspoon ground turmeric

- 1 teaspoon ground cumin

- 1 teaspoon ground coriander

- Salt and pepper to taste

- Fresh cilantro for garnish

Instructions:

1. In a large pot, combine red lentils, coconut milk, vegetable broth, diced onion, minced garlic, curry powder, turmeric, cumin, coriander, salt, and pepper.

2. Bring the mixture to a boil, then reduce heat and let it simmer for 20-25 minutes, or until the lentils are soft and cooked through.

3. Taste and adjust seasoning if needed.

4. Serve hot, garnished with fresh cilantro.

5. Enjoy this creamy and aromatic coconut curry lentil soup.

16.Grilled Lemon Herb Chicken

Ingredients:

- 4 boneless, skinless chicken breasts

- Zest and juice of 1 lemon

- 2 cloves garlic, minced

- 2 tablespoons chopped fresh herbs (such as parsley, thyme, or rosemary)

- 2 tablespoons olive oil

- Salt and pepper to taste

Instructions:

1. In a bowl, whisk together lemon zest, lemon juice, minced garlic, chopped fresh herbs, olive oil, salt, and pepper to make a marinade.

2. Place chicken breasts in a shallow dish and pour the marinade over them. Ensure the chicken is evenly coated. Cover and refrigerate for at least 30 minutes, or up to 4 hours.

3. Preheat grill to medium-high heat.

4. Remove chicken from marinade and discard excess marinade.

5. Grill chicken for 6-8 minutes per side, or until cooked through and no longer pink in the center.

6. Let the chicken rest for a few minutes before slicing.

7. Serve hot with your favorite side dishes for a delicious and protein-packed meal.

17.Mediterranean Quinoa Salad

Ingredients:

- 1 cup quinoa, rinsed

- 2 cups water or vegetable broth

- 1 cucumber, diced

- 1 bell pepper, diced

- 1 cup cherry tomatoes, halved

- 1/4 cup red onion, finely chopped

- 1/4 cup Kalamata olives, pitted and chopped

- 1/4 cup crumbled feta cheese

- 1/4 cup chopped fresh parsley

- 2 tablespoons extra virgin olive oil

- 2 tablespoons lemon juice

- 1 teaspoon dried oregano

- Salt and pepper to taste

Instructions:

1. In a medium saucepan, bring water or vegetable broth to a boil. Add quinoa, reduce heat to low, cover, and simmer for 15-20 minutes, or until quinoa is cooked and liquid is absorbed. Remove from heat and let it cool.

2. In a large bowl, combine cooked quinoa, diced cucumber, bell pepper, cherry tomatoes, red onion, Kalamata olives, crumbled feta cheese, and chopped parsley.

3. In a small bowl, whisk together extra virgin olive oil, lemon juice, dried oregano, salt, and pepper to make the dressing.

4. Pour the dressing over the quinoa salad and toss until everything is well combined.

5. Taste and adjust seasoning if needed.

6. Serve chilled or at room temperature as a refreshing and nutritious salad.

18.Butternut Squash and Apple Soup

Ingredients:

- 1 medium butternut squash, peeled, seeded, and diced

- 2 apples, peeled, cored, and diced

- 1 onion, diced

- 2 cloves garlic, minced

- 4 cups vegetable broth

- 1 teaspoon ground cinnamon

- 1/2 teaspoon ground nutmeg

- Salt and pepper to taste

- 2 tablespoons olive oil

- Optional toppings: toasted pumpkin seeds, Greek yogurt, chopped fresh herbs

Instructions:

1. In a large pot, heat olive oil over medium heat. Add diced onion and minced garlic. Sauté until onions are translucent.

2. Add diced butternut squash and apples to the pot. Cook for 5-7 minutes, stirring occasionally.

3. Pour in vegetable broth and bring to a boil. Reduce heat to low, cover, and simmer for 20-25 minutes, or until the squash and apples are tender.

4. Use an immersion blender or transfer the soup to a blender to puree until smooth.

5. Stir in ground cinnamon and nutmeg. Season with salt and pepper to taste.

6. Serve hot, garnished with optional toppings such as toasted pumpkin seeds, a dollop of Greek yogurt, or chopped fresh herbs.

7. Enjoy this comforting and flavorful butternut squash and apple soup.

19.Roasted Beet and Goat Cheese Salad

Ingredients:

- 4 medium beets, peeled and diced

- 2 tablespoons olive oil

- Salt and pepper to taste

- 4 cups mixed salad greens

- 1/2 cup crumbled goat cheese

- 1/4 cup chopped walnuts or pecans

- Balsamic glaze for drizzling

Instructions:

1. Preheat the oven to 400°F (200°C).

2. Place diced beets on a baking sheet lined with parchment paper. Drizzle with olive oil, and season with salt and pepper. Toss to coat evenly.

3. Roast beets in the preheated oven for 25-30 minutes, or until tender and slightly caramelized, stirring halfway through.

4. Arrange mixed salad greens on a serving platter.

5. Top with roasted beets, crumbled goat cheese, and chopped walnuts or pecans.

6. Drizzle with balsamic glaze just before serving.

7. Enjoy this vibrant and flavorful roasted beet and goat cheese salad as a light and nutritious meal.

20. Sautéed Garlic Shrimp with Lemon and Parsley

Ingredients:

- 1 pound large shrimp, peeled and deveined

- 3 cloves garlic, minced

- 2 tablespoons olive oil

- Juice of 1 lemon

- Zest of 1 lemon

- 2 tablespoons chopped fresh parsley

- Salt and pepper to taste

Instructions:

1. Heat olive oil in a large skillet over medium heat.

2. Add minced garlic to the skillet and sauté for 1-2 minutes, until fragrant.

3. Add shrimp to the skillet in a single layer. Cook for 2-3 minutes on each side, or until shrimp are pink and opaque.

4. Season shrimp with salt, pepper, lemon juice, lemon zest, and chopped parsley.

5. Toss shrimp in the skillet to coat evenly with the garlic, lemon, and parsley mixture.

6. Remove from heat and transfer shrimp to a serving plate.

7. Serve hot as an appetizer or main dish, garnished with additional parsley if desired.

21.Baked Salmon with Honey Mustard Glaze

Ingredients:

- 4 salmon fillets

- 3 tablespoons Dijon mustard

- 2 tablespoons honey

- 1 tablespoon soy sauce

- 2 cloves garlic, minced

- Salt and pepper to taste

- Lemon wedges for serving

Instructions:

1. Preheat the oven to 375°F (190°C).

2. In a small bowl, whisk together Dijon mustard, honey, soy sauce, minced garlic, salt, and pepper to make the glaze.

3. Place salmon fillets on a baking sheet lined with parchment paper.

4. Brush the salmon fillets with the honey mustard glaze, coating them evenly.

5. Bake in the preheated oven for 12-15 minutes, or until the salmon is cooked through and flakes easily with a fork.

6. Serve hot, with lemon wedges on the side for squeezing over the salmon.

22.Greek Chicken Gyros with Tzatziki Sauce

Ingredients:

For the chicken marinade:

- 1 pound boneless, skinless chicken breasts, sliced into strips

- 2 tablespoons Greek yogurt

- 2 tablespoons olive oil

- Juice of 1 lemon

- 2 cloves garlic, minced

- 1 teaspoon dried oregano

- Salt and pepper to taste

For the tzatziki sauce:

- 1 cup Greek yogurt

- 1 cucumber, grated and squeezed to remove excess moisture

- 2 cloves garlic, minced

- 1 tablespoon lemon juice

- 1 tablespoon chopped fresh dill

- Salt and pepper to taste

Instructions:

1. In a bowl, combine Greek yogurt, olive oil, lemon juice, minced garlic, dried oregano, salt, and pepper to make the chicken marinade.

2. Add sliced chicken breasts to the marinade and toss to coat evenly. Cover and refrigerate for at least 30 minutes, or up to 4 hours.

3. In another bowl, mix together Greek yogurt, grated cucumber, minced garlic, lemon juice, chopped fresh dill, salt, and pepper to make the tzatziki sauce. Cover and refrigerate until ready to use.

4. Preheat a grill or grill pan over medium-high heat. Thread marinated chicken strips onto skewers and grill for 4-5 minutes on each side, or until cooked through and lightly charred.

5. Warm pitas or flatbreads on the grill for a minute on each side.

6. Assemble gyros by placing grilled chicken strips on warmed pitas, and topping with tzatziki sauce, sliced tomatoes, onions, and lettuce.

7. Serve immediately, with additional tzatziki sauce on the side for dipping.

23.Vegetable Stir-Fry with Tofu

Ingredients:

- 1 block firm tofu, pressed and cubed

- 2 tablespoons soy sauce

- 1 tablespoon sesame oil

- 1 tablespoon cornstarch

- 2 tablespoons vegetable oil

- 2 cups mixed vegetables (such as bell peppers, broccoli, carrots, and snap peas), chopped

- 3 cloves garlic, minced

- 1 tablespoon minced ginger

- Cooked rice or noodles for serving

Instructions:

1. In a bowl, combine cubed tofu with soy sauce, sesame oil, and cornstarch. Toss to coat evenly and let it marinate for 10-15 minutes.

2. Heat vegetable oil in a large skillet or wok over medium-high heat. Add marinated tofu cubes and cook until golden brown and crispy on all sides. Remove tofu from the skillet and set aside.

3. In the same skillet, add more vegetable oil if needed. Add minced garlic and ginger, and stir-fry for 1-2 minutes until fragrant.

4. Add chopped mixed vegetables to the skillet and stir-fry for 4-5 minutes, or until vegetables are tender-crisp.

5. Return cooked tofu to the skillet and toss to combine with the vegetables.

6. Serve hot over cooked rice or noodles for a satisfying and nutritious meal.

24.Quinoa Stuffed Bell Peppers

Ingredients:

- 4 large bell peppers, halved and seeds removed

- 1 cup quinoa, rinsed

- 2 cups vegetable broth

- 1 can black beans, drained and rinsed

- 1 cup corn kernels (fresh, canned, or frozen)

- 1 cup diced tomatoes

- 1 teaspoon ground cumin

- 1 teaspoon chili powder

- Salt and pepper to taste

- 1/2 cup shredded cheese (such as cheddar or Monterey Jack)

- Chopped fresh cilantro for garnish

Instructions:

1. Preheat the oven to 375°F (190°C).

2. In a medium saucepan, bring vegetable broth to a boil. Add quinoa, reduce heat to low, cover, and simmer for 15-20 minutes, or until quinoa is cooked and liquid is absorbed.

3. In a large bowl, combine cooked quinoa, black beans, corn kernels, diced tomatoes, ground cumin, chili powder, salt, and pepper.

4. Fill each bell pepper half with the quinoa mixture and place them in a baking dish.

5. Cover the baking dish with aluminum foil and bake in the preheated oven for 25-30 minutes, or until bell peppers are tender.

6. Remove the foil, sprinkle shredded cheese on top of each stuffed bell pepper, and return to the oven. Bake for an additional 5 minutes, or until the cheese is melted and bubbly.

7. Garnish with chopped fresh cilantro before serving.

25.Berry Chia Seed Pudding

Ingredients:

- 1/4 cup chia seeds

- 1 cup unsweetened almond milk (or any milk of your choice)

- 1 tablespoon honey or maple syrup (optional)

- 1/2 teaspoon vanilla extract

- 1 cup mixed berries (such as strawberries, blueberries, and raspberries)

- Additional berries and mint leaves for garnish

Instructions:

1. In a bowl, whisk together chia seeds, almond milk, honey or maple syrup (if using), and vanilla extract.

2. Let the mixture sit for 5-10 minutes, then whisk again to break up any clumps of chia seeds.

3. Cover the bowl and refrigerate for at least 2 hours, or overnight, until the chia pudding has thickened.

4. Before serving, stir the chia pudding to ensure an even consistency.

5. In serving glasses or bowls, layer the chia pudding with mixed berries.

6. Garnish with additional berries and mint leaves.

7. Serve chilled as a nutritious and delicious dessert or breakfast option.

26. Turkey and Vegetable Meatball Soup

Ingredients:

- 1 pound ground turkey
- 1/4 cup breadcrumbs
- 1 egg
- 1/4 cup grated Parmesan cheese
- 1/2 teaspoon garlic powder
- 1/2 teaspoon dried oregano
- Salt and pepper to taste
- 1 tablespoon olive oil
- 1 onion, diced
- 2 carrots, diced
- 2 celery stalks, diced
- 2 cloves garlic, minced
- 6 cups low-sodium chicken broth
- 1 can diced tomatoes

- 2 cups chopped spinach or kale

- 1/4 cup chopped fresh parsley

- Cooked pasta or rice for serving

Instructions:

1. In a large bowl, combine ground turkey, breadcrumbs, egg, Parmesan cheese, garlic powder, dried oregano, salt, and pepper. Mix until well combined, then shape the mixture into small meatballs.

2. Heat olive oil in a large pot over medium heat. Add meatballs and cook until browned on all sides. Remove meatballs from the pot and set aside.

3. In the same pot, add diced onion, carrots, celery, and minced garlic. Sauté until vegetables are softened.

4. Pour in chicken broth and diced tomatoes with their juices. Bring the mixture to a simmer.

5. Add cooked meatballs back to the pot and let the soup simmer for 15-20 minutes.

6. Stir in chopped spinach or kale and chopped fresh parsley. Cook for an additional 5 minutes until greens are wilted.

7. Taste and adjust seasoning if needed.

8. Serve hot over cooked pasta or rice for a comforting and hearty meal.

27.Roasted Brussels Sprouts with Balsamic Glaze

Ingredients:

- 1 pound Brussels sprouts, trimmed and halved

- 2 tablespoons olive oil

- Salt and pepper to taste

- 2 tablespoons balsamic vinegar

- 1 tablespoon honey or maple syrup (optional)

- 2 tablespoons chopped toasted pecans or walnuts (optional)

Instructions:

1. Preheat the oven to 400°F (200°C).

2. In a large bowl, toss Brussels sprouts with olive oil, salt, and pepper until evenly coated.

3. Spread Brussels sprouts in a single layer on a baking sheet lined with parchment paper.

4. Roast in the preheated oven for 25-30 minutes, or until Brussels sprouts are golden brown and crispy on the edges, stirring halfway through.

5. In a small saucepan, combine balsamic vinegar and honey or maple syrup (if using). Bring to a simmer and cook for 2-3 minutes, or until the glaze has thickened slightly.

6. Drizzle the balsamic glaze over the roasted Brussels sprouts just before serving.

7. Sprinkle with chopped toasted pecans or walnuts if desired.

8. Serve hot as a flavorful and nutritious side dish.

28. Mediterranean Chickpea Salad

Ingredients:

- 2 cans chickpeas, drained and rinsed
- 1 cucumber, diced
- 1 bell pepper, diced
- 1/4 cup diced red onion
- 1/4 cup chopped fresh parsley
- 1/4 cup crumbled feta cheese
- 2 tablespoons extra virgin olive oil
- 2 tablespoons lemon juice
- 1 teaspoon dried oregano
- Salt and pepper to taste

Instructions:

1. In a large bowl, combine chickpeas, diced cucumber, diced bell pepper, diced red onion, chopped fresh parsley, and crumbled feta cheese.

2. In a small bowl, whisk together extra virgin olive oil, lemon juice, dried oregano, salt, and pepper to make the dressing.

3. Pour the dressing over the chickpea salad and toss until everything is well combined.

4. Taste and adjust seasoning if needed.

5. Serve chilled or at room temperature as a refreshing and protein-rich salad.

29. Lemon Garlic Butter Pasta with Shrimp

Ingredients:

- 8 ounces pasta (linguine or spaghetti)
- 1 pound large shrimp, peeled and deveined
- Salt and pepper to taste
- 3 tablespoons unsalted butter
- 4 cloves garlic, minced
- Zest and juice of 1 lemon
- 1/4 cup chopped fresh parsley

- Grated Parmesan cheese for serving (optional)

Instructions:

1. Cook pasta according to package instructions until al dente. Drain and set aside, reserving some pasta water.

2. Season shrimp with salt and pepper to taste.

3. In a large skillet, melt butter over medium heat. Add minced garlic and cook until fragrant, about 1 minute.

4. Add seasoned shrimp to the skillet and cook for 2-3 minutes on each side, until pink and cooked through. Remove shrimp from the skillet and set aside.

5. In the same skillet, add cooked pasta along with lemon zest and lemon juice. Toss to coat the pasta with the lemon garlic butter sauce. If the sauce is too thick, add a splash of reserved pasta water to loosen it up.

6. Add cooked shrimp back to the skillet and toss with the pasta.

7. Sprinkle chopped fresh parsley over the pasta and shrimp.

8. Serve hot, optionally garnished with grated Parmesan cheese, for a delicious and satisfying meal.

30. Hearty Minestrone Soup

Ingredients:

- 2 tablespoons olive oil

- 1 onion, diced

- 2 carrots, diced

- 2 celery stalks, diced

- 2 cloves garlic, minced

- 1 can diced tomatoes

- 6 cups vegetable broth

- 1 cup small pasta (such as ditalini or elbow macaroni)

- 1 can kidney beans, drained and rinsed

- 1 can cannellini beans, drained and rinsed

- 1 cup chopped spinach or kale

- 1 teaspoon dried oregano

- 1 teaspoon dried basil

- Salt and pepper to taste

- Grated Parmesan cheese for serving (optional)

Instructions:

1. In a large pot, heat olive oil over medium heat. Add diced onion, carrots, and celery. Sauté until vegetables are softened.

2. Add minced garlic to the pot and cook for another minute until fragrant.

3. Stir in diced tomatoes, vegetable broth, small pasta, kidney beans, cannellini beans, dried oregano, dried basil, salt, and pepper.

4. Bring the soup to a boil, then reduce heat to low and let it simmer for 15-20 minutes, or until pasta is cooked and vegetables are tender.

5. Stir in chopped spinach or kale and cook for an additional 5 minutes.

6. Taste and adjust seasoning if needed.

7. Serve hot, optionally garnished with grated Parmesan cheese, for a comforting and nutritious meal.

31.Grilled Vegetable Platter

Ingredients:

- Assorted vegetables (such as bell peppers, zucchini, eggplant, mushrooms, and cherry tomatoes), sliced

- 2 tablespoons olive oil

- Salt and pepper to taste

- Balsamic glaze for drizzling

- Fresh herbs for garnish (such as basil or parsley)

Instructions:

1. Preheat grill to medium-high heat.

2. In a large bowl, toss sliced vegetables with olive oil, salt, and pepper until evenly coated.

3. Arrange vegetables on the preheated grill. Grill for 4-5 minutes on each side, or until tender and lightly charred.

4. Transfer grilled vegetables to a serving platter.

5. Drizzle with balsamic glaze and garnish with fresh herbs.

6. Serve hot or at room temperature as a colorful and flavorful side dish or appetizer.

32.Baked Stuffed Portobello Mushrooms

Ingredients:

- 4 large portobello mushrooms, stems removed

- 1 cup cooked quinoa or brown rice

- 1 cup chopped spinach

- 1/2 cup diced bell pepper

- 1/4 cup diced red onion

- 2 cloves garlic, minced

- 1/4 cup grated Parmesan cheese

- 2 tablespoons olive oil

- 1 teaspoon dried Italian herbs (such as oregano, basil, and thyme)

- Salt and pepper to taste

- 1/4 cup shredded mozzarella cheese (optional)

Instructions:

1. Preheat the oven to 375°F (190°C).

2. Place portobello mushrooms on a baking sheet lined with parchment paper, gill side up.

3. In a skillet, heat olive oil over medium heat. Add minced garlic, diced bell pepper, and diced red onion. Sauté until vegetables are softened.

4. Add chopped spinach to the skillet and cook until wilted.

5. Stir in cooked quinoa or brown rice, grated Parmesan cheese, dried Italian herbs, salt, and pepper. Cook for another 2-3 minutes to combine flavors.

6. Spoon the quinoa mixture into each portobello mushroom cap, pressing down gently to pack it in.

7. If desired, sprinkle shredded mozzarella cheese on top of each stuffed mushroom.

8. Bake in the preheated oven for 20-25 minutes, or until mushrooms are tender and filling is heated through.

9. Serve hot as a satisfying and flavorful vegetarian main dish.

33.Honey Garlic Glazed Salmon

Ingredients:

- 4 salmon fillets

- 3 tablespoons honey

- 2 tablespoons soy sauce

- 2 cloves garlic, minced

- 1 tablespoon olive oil

- Salt and pepper to taste

- Sesame seeds and chopped green onions for garnish (optional)

Instructions:

1. In a bowl, whisk together honey, soy sauce, minced garlic, olive oil, salt, and pepper to make the glaze.

2. Place salmon fillets in a shallow dish and pour the honey garlic glaze over them. Ensure the salmon is evenly coated. Let it marinate for 15-20 minutes.

3. Preheat the oven to 400°F (200°C).

4. Heat a skillet over medium-high heat. Add marinated salmon fillets to the skillet, skin side down, and cook for 2-3 minutes until golden brown.

5. Transfer the skillet to the preheated oven and bake for 10-12 minutes, or until salmon is cooked through and flakes easily with a fork.

6. Serve hot, garnished with sesame seeds and chopped green onions if desired.

34. Quinoa and Black Bean Stuffed Bell Peppers

Ingredients:

- 4 large bell peppers, halved and seeds removed

- 1 cup cooked quinoa

- 1 can black beans, drained and rinsed

- 1 cup corn kernels (fresh, canned, or frozen)

- 1 cup diced tomatoes

- 1 teaspoon ground cumin

- 1 teaspoon chili powder

- Salt and pepper to taste

- 1/2 cup shredded cheddar cheese

- Fresh cilantro for garnish

Instructions:

1. Preheat the oven to 375°F (190°C).

2. In a large bowl, combine cooked quinoa, black beans, corn kernels, diced tomatoes, ground cumin, chili powder, salt, and pepper.

3. Fill each bell pepper half with the quinoa mixture and place them in a baking dish.

4. Cover the baking dish with aluminum foil and bake in the preheated oven for 25-30 minutes, or until bell peppers are tender.

5. Remove the foil, sprinkle shredded cheddar cheese on top of each stuffed bell pepper, and return to the oven. Bake for an additional 5 minutes, or until the cheese is melted and bubbly.

6. Garnish with fresh cilantro before serving.

35.Mediterranean Lentil Salad

Ingredients:

- 1 cup dried lentils

- 2 cups water

- 1 cucumber, diced

- 1 bell pepper, diced

- 1/4 cup red onion, finely chopped

- 1/4 cup Kalamata olives, pitted and chopped

- 1/4 cup crumbled feta cheese

- 2 tablespoons chopped fresh parsley

- 2 tablespoons extra virgin olive oil

- 2 tablespoons lemon juice

- 1 teaspoon dried oregano

- Salt and pepper to taste

Instructions:

1. Rinse the lentils under cold water. In a pot, combine the lentils and water. Bring to a boil, then reduce heat to low and simmer for 20-25 minutes, or until lentils are tender but still hold their shape. Drain any excess water and let the lentils cool.

2. In a large bowl, combine the cooked lentils, diced cucumber, diced bell pepper, finely chopped red onion, chopped Kalamata olives, crumbled feta cheese, and chopped fresh parsley.

3. In a small bowl, whisk together the extra virgin olive oil, lemon juice, dried oregano, salt, and pepper to make the dressing.

4. Pour the dressing over the lentil salad and toss until everything is well coated.

5. Taste and adjust seasoning if needed.

6. Serve chilled or at room temperature as a refreshing and nutritious salad.

36. Baked Chicken Parmesan

Ingredients:

- 4 boneless, skinless chicken breasts
- Salt and pepper to taste
- 1/2 cup all-purpose flour
- 2 eggs, beaten
- 1 cup breadcrumbs
- 1/2 cup grated Parmesan cheese
- 2 cups marinara sauce

- 1 cup shredded mozzarella cheese

- Fresh basil leaves for garnish (optional)

Instructions:

1. Preheat the oven to 400°F (200°C). Lightly grease a baking dish.

2. Season chicken breasts with salt and pepper to taste.

3. Set up a breading station: Place flour in one shallow dish, beaten eggs in another dish, and breadcrumbs mixed with grated Parmesan cheese in a third dish.

4. Dredge each chicken breast in flour, then dip into beaten eggs, and coat with breadcrumb mixture, pressing gently to adhere.

5. Place breaded chicken breasts in the prepared baking dish. Bake in the preheated oven for 20-25 minutes, or until chicken is cooked through and golden brown.

6. Remove chicken from the oven and spoon marinara sauce over each breast. Sprinkle shredded mozzarella cheese on top.

7. Return the baking dish to the oven and bake for an additional 5-10 minutes, or until cheese is melted and bubbly.

8. Garnish with fresh basil leaves before serving.

37. Lemon Herb Roasted Vegetables

Ingredients:

- Assorted vegetables (such as carrots, potatoes, Brussels sprouts, and cauliflower), cut into bite-sized pieces

- 2 tablespoons olive oil

- Zest and juice of 1 lemon

- 2 cloves garlic, minced

- 1 teaspoon dried thyme

- 1 teaspoon dried rosemary

- Salt and pepper to taste

- Fresh parsley for garnish (optional)

Instructions:

1. Preheat the oven to 400°F (200°C).

2. In a large bowl, toss together the assorted vegetables, olive oil, lemon zest, lemon juice, minced garlic, dried thyme, dried rosemary, salt, and pepper until well coated.

3. Spread the seasoned vegetables in a single layer on a baking sheet lined with parchment paper.

4. Roast in the preheated oven for 25-30 minutes, or until vegetables are tender and caramelized, stirring halfway through.

5. Garnish with fresh parsley before serving.

38.Spinach and Feta Stuffed Chicken Breast

Ingredients:

- 4 boneless, skinless chicken breasts

- Salt and pepper to taste

- 2 cups fresh spinach leaves

- 1/2 cup crumbled feta cheese

- 2 cloves garlic, minced

- 1 tablespoon olive oil

- 1 teaspoon dried oregano

- Toothpicks or kitchen twine

Instructions:

1. Preheat the oven to 375°F (190°C). Lightly grease a baking dish.

2. Season chicken breasts with salt and pepper.

3. In a skillet, heat olive oil over medium heat. Add minced garlic and cook until fragrant, about 1 minute.

4. Add fresh spinach leaves to the skillet and cook until wilted. Remove from heat and let it cool slightly.

5. Once cooled, squeeze excess moisture from the spinach and transfer it to a bowl. Stir in crumbled feta cheese and dried oregano.

6. Make a horizontal slit in each chicken breast to create a pocket without cutting all the way through.

7. Stuff each chicken breast with the spinach and feta mixture, then secure the openings with toothpicks or kitchen twine.

8. Place stuffed chicken breasts in the prepared baking dish.

9. Bake in the preheated oven for 25-30 minutes, or until chicken is cooked through and juices run clear.

10. Remove toothpicks or twine before serving.

39.Quinoa and Vegetable Stir-Fry

Ingredients:

- 1 cup quinoa, rinsed

- 2 cups water or vegetable broth

- 2 tablespoons soy sauce

- 1 tablespoon sesame oil

- 1 tablespoon olive oil

- 2 cloves garlic, minced

- 1 bell pepper, sliced

- 1 carrot, julienned

- 1 cup broccoli florets

- 1 cup snap peas

- Salt and pepper to taste

- Sesame seeds for garnish (optional)

- Chopped green onions for garnish (optional)

Instructions:

1. In a saucepan, combine quinoa and water or vegetable broth. Bring to a boil, then reduce heat to low, cover, and simmer for 15-20 minutes, or until quinoa is cooked and liquid is absorbed.

Remove from heat and let it sit for 5 minutes before fluffing with a fork.

2. In a small bowl, whisk together soy sauce and sesame oil to make the sauce.

3. Heat olive oil in a large skillet or wok over medium-high heat. Add minced garlic and cook until fragrant, about 1 minute.

4. Add sliced bell pepper, julienned carrot, broccoli florets, and snap peas to the skillet. Stir-fry for 4-5 minutes, or until vegetables are tender-crisp.

5. Add cooked quinoa to the skillet, then pour the sauce over the quinoa and vegetables. Toss everything together until well combined and heated through.

6. Season with salt and pepper to taste.

7. Garnish with sesame seeds and chopped green onions before serving.

40.Greek Yogurt Parfait with Berries and Granola

Ingredients:

- 2 cups Greek yogurt

- 1 cup mixed berries (such as strawberries, blueberries, and raspberries)

- 1/2 cup granola

- Honey or maple syrup for drizzling (optional)

Instructions:

1. In serving glasses or bowls, layer Greek yogurt, mixed berries, and granola.

2. Drizzle with honey or maple syrup if desired.

3. Serve immediately as a nutritious and delicious breakfast or snack option.

41. Lemon Garlic Roasted Chicken Thighs

Ingredients:

- 6 chicken thighs, bone-in and skin-on
- Salt and pepper to taste
- 2 tablespoons olive oil
- 4 cloves garlic, minced
- Zest and juice of 1 lemon
- 1 teaspoon dried thyme
- 1 teaspoon dried rosemary
- Fresh parsley for garnish (optional)

Instructions:

1. Preheat the oven to 400°F (200°C). Lightly grease a baking dish.

2. Pat dry the chicken thighs with paper towels and season them generously with salt and pepper.

3. In a small bowl, whisk together olive oil, minced garlic, lemon zest, lemon juice, dried thyme, and dried rosemary.

4. Place the chicken thighs in the prepared baking dish and pour the lemon garlic mixture over them, ensuring they are evenly coated.

5. Arrange the chicken thighs skin side up in the baking dish.

6. Roast in the preheated oven for 30-35 minutes, or until the chicken is golden brown and cooked through, with juices running clear.

7. Garnish with fresh parsley before serving.

42. Mediterranean Quinoa Salad

Ingredients:

- 1 cup quinoa, rinsed
- 2 cups water or vegetable broth
- 1 cucumber, diced
- 1 bell pepper, diced
- 1/4 cup red onion, finely chopped
- 1/4 cup Kalamata olives, pitted and chopped
- 1/4 cup crumbled feta cheese
- 2 tablespoons chopped fresh parsley
- 2 tablespoons extra virgin olive oil
- 2 tablespoons lemon juice
- 1 teaspoon dried oregano

- Salt and pepper to taste

Instructions:

1. In a saucepan, combine quinoa and water or vegetable broth. Bring to a boil, then reduce heat to low, cover, and simmer for 15-20 minutes, or until quinoa is cooked and liquid is absorbed. Remove from heat and let it cool.

2. In a large bowl, combine cooked quinoa, diced cucumber, diced bell pepper, finely chopped red onion, chopped Kalamata olives, crumbled feta cheese, and chopped fresh parsley.

3. In a small bowl, whisk together extra virgin olive oil, lemon juice, dried oregano, salt, and pepper to make the dressing.

4. Pour the dressing over the quinoa salad and toss until everything is well coated.

5. Taste and adjust seasoning if needed.

6. Serve chilled or at room temperature as a refreshing and nutritious salad.

43. Roasted Sweet Potatoes with Honey and Cinnamon

Ingredients:

- 2 large sweet potatoes, peeled and cut into cubes

- 2 tablespoons olive oil

- 2 tablespoons honey

- 1 teaspoon ground cinnamon

- Salt to taste

- Chopped fresh parsley for garnish (optional)

Instructions:

1. Preheat the oven to 400°F (200°C). Line a baking sheet with parchment paper.

2. In a large bowl, toss sweet potato cubes with olive oil, honey, ground cinnamon, and salt until evenly coated.

3. Spread the sweet potato cubes in a single layer on the prepared baking sheet.

4. Roast in the preheated oven for 25-30 minutes, or until sweet potatoes are tender and caramelized, stirring halfway through.

5. Garnish with chopped fresh parsley before serving.

44.Lemon Herb Grilled Chicken Breast

Ingredients:

- 4 boneless, skinless chicken breasts

- Salt and pepper to taste

- Zest and juice of 1 lemon

- 2 tablespoons olive oil

- 2 cloves garlic, minced

- 1 teaspoon dried oregano

- 1 teaspoon dried thyme

- Fresh parsley for garnish (optional)

Instructions:

1. Season chicken breasts with salt and pepper on both sides.

2. In a bowl, whisk together lemon zest, lemon juice, olive oil, minced garlic, dried oregano, and dried thyme to make the marinade.

3. Place chicken breasts in a shallow dish or resealable plastic bag. Pour the marinade over the chicken, ensuring each piece is well coated. Marinate in the refrigerator for at least 30 minutes, or up to 4 hours.

4. Preheat grill to medium-high heat.

5. Remove chicken breasts from the marinade and discard any excess marinade.

6. Grill chicken breasts for 6-8 minutes per side, or until cooked through and juices run clear.

7. Remove from the grill and let the chicken rest for a few minutes before serving.

8. Garnish with fresh parsley before serving.

45. Butternut Squash Soup

Ingredients:

- 1 medium butternut squash, peeled, seeded, and diced

- 1 onion, diced

- 2 carrots, diced

- 2 stalks celery, diced

- 4 cups vegetable broth

- 1 teaspoon dried thyme

- 1/2 teaspoon ground cinnamon

- Salt and pepper to taste

- 1/4 cup heavy cream (optional)

- Toasted pumpkin seeds for garnish (optional)

- Chopped fresh parsley for garnish (optional)

Instructions:

1. In a large pot, combine diced butternut squash, diced onion, diced carrots, diced celery, vegetable broth, dried thyme, and ground cinnamon.

2. Bring the mixture to a boil, then reduce heat to low and simmer for 20-25 minutes, or until vegetables are tender.

3. Use an immersion blender to puree the soup until smooth. Alternatively, transfer the soup in batches to a blender and blend until smooth. Be cautious when blending hot liquids.

4. Season the soup with salt and pepper to taste. Stir in heavy cream if using, then simmer for an additional 5 minutes.

5. Serve hot, garnished with toasted pumpkin seeds and chopped fresh parsley if desired.

46. Oven-Roasted Brussels Sprouts with Balsamic Glaze

Ingredients:

- 1 pound Brussels sprouts, trimmed and halved

- 2 tablespoons olive oil

- Salt and pepper to taste

- 2 tablespoons balsamic vinegar

- 1 tablespoon honey or maple syrup

- 1/4 cup grated Parmesan cheese (optional)

- Chopped fresh parsley for garnish (optional)

Instructions:

1. Preheat the oven to 400°F (200°C). Line a baking sheet with parchment paper.

2. In a large bowl, toss Brussels sprouts with olive oil, salt, and pepper until evenly coated.

3. Spread Brussels sprouts in a single layer on the prepared baking sheet.

4. Roast in the preheated oven for 25-30 minutes, or until Brussels sprouts are tender and caramelized, stirring halfway through.

5. In a small saucepan, combine balsamic vinegar and honey or maple syrup. Bring to a simmer and cook

for 2-3 minutes, or until the glaze has thickened slightly.

6. Drizzle the balsamic glaze over the roasted Brussels sprouts just before serving.

7. Optional: Sprinkle with grated Parmesan cheese and chopped fresh parsley for extra flavor.

47. Lemon Garlic Shrimp Scampi

Ingredients:

- 1 pound shrimp, peeled and deveined
- Salt and pepper to taste
- 8 ounces linguine or spaghetti
- 3 tablespoons unsalted butter
- 4 cloves garlic, minced
- Zest and juice of 1 lemon
- 1/4 cup dry white wine or chicken broth
- 1/4 cup chopped fresh parsley
- Grated Parmesan cheese for serving (optional)

Instructions:

1. Season shrimp with salt and pepper to taste.

2. Cook pasta according to package instructions until al dente. Drain and set aside.

3. In a large skillet, melt butter over medium heat. Add minced garlic and cook until fragrant, about 1 minute.

4. Add seasoned shrimp to the skillet and cook for 2-3 minutes on each side, until pink and cooked through. Remove shrimp from the skillet and set aside.

5. Deglaze the skillet with dry white wine or chicken broth, scraping up any browned bits from the bottom of the pan.

6. Stir in lemon zest and lemon juice, then add cooked pasta to the skillet. Toss to coat the pasta with the lemon garlic sauce.

7. Return cooked shrimp to the skillet and toss with the pasta.

8. Sprinkle chopped fresh parsley over the shrimp scampi.

9. Serve hot, optionally garnished with grated Parmesan cheese, for a delicious and satisfying meal.

48.Avocado and Black Bean Quesadillas

Ingredients:

- 4 large flour tortillas

- 1 ripe avocado, mashed

- 1 cup canned black beans, drained and rinsed

- 1 cup shredded Monterey Jack cheese

- 1/2 cup salsa

- 2 tablespoons chopped fresh cilantro

- 1 tablespoon olive oil

Instructions:

1. Spread mashed avocado evenly onto one half of each tortilla.

2. Top the avocado with black beans, shredded Monterey Jack cheese, salsa, and chopped fresh cilantro.

3. Fold the tortillas in half to enclose the filling, creating quesadillas.

4. Heat olive oil in a large skillet over medium heat. Place the quesadillas in the skillet and cook for 2-3 minutes on each side, or until golden brown and crispy, and the cheese is melted.

5. Remove from the skillet and let them cool for a minute before slicing into wedges.

6. Serve hot as a tasty and satisfying meal or snack.

49.Greek Yogurt Chicken Salad

Ingredients:

- 2 cups cooked chicken, shredded or diced

- 1/2 cup Greek yogurt

- 2 tablespoons mayonnaise

- 1 tablespoon Dijon mustard

- 1 celery stalk, finely chopped

- 1/4 cup red onion, finely chopped

- 1/4 cup chopped fresh parsley

- Salt and pepper to taste

- Lettuce leaves or bread for serving

Instructions:

1. In a large bowl, combine cooked chicken, Greek yogurt, mayonnaise, Dijon mustard, chopped celery, chopped red onion, and chopped fresh parsley.

2. Season with salt and pepper to taste and mix until well combined.

3. Serve the chicken salad over lettuce leaves as a light and refreshing salad, or spread it between slices of bread to make sandwiches.

4. Enjoy as a nutritious and satisfying meal.

50. Vegetarian Lentil Curry

Ingredients:

- 1 cup dried lentils

- 3 cups vegetable broth

- 1 onion, diced

- 2 cloves garlic, minced

- 1 tablespoon grated fresh ginger

- 1 bell pepper, diced

- 1 carrot, diced

- 1 tablespoon curry powder

- 1 teaspoon ground cumin

- 1 teaspoon ground coriander

- 1/2 teaspoon turmeric

- 1 can (14 ounces) diced tomatoes

- 1 can (14 ounces) coconut milk

- Salt and pepper to taste

- Fresh cilantro for garnish (optional)

- Cooked rice for serving

Instructions:

1. Rinse the lentils under cold water. In a pot, combine lentils and vegetable broth. Bring to a boil, then reduce heat to low, cover, and simmer for 20-25 minutes, or until lentils are tender.

2. In a separate large skillet, heat some oil over medium heat. Add diced onion, minced garlic, and grated ginger. Sauté until fragrant and onions are translucent.

3. Add diced bell pepper and diced carrot to the skillet. Cook until vegetables are slightly softened.

4. Stir in curry powder, ground cumin, ground coriander, and turmeric. Cook for another minute to toast the spices.

5. Add diced tomatoes (with their juices) and coconut milk to the skillet. Stir to combine.

6. Once the lentils are cooked, add them to the skillet with the vegetable-coconut milk mixture. Season with salt and pepper to taste.

7. Let the curry simmer for 10-15 minutes to allow the flavors to meld together and the sauce to thicken.

8. Taste and adjust seasoning if needed.

9. Serve hot over cooked rice, garnished with fresh cilantro if desired.

51.Roasted Vegetable and Hummus Wraps

Ingredients:

- Assorted vegetables (such as bell peppers, zucchini, eggplant, and red onion), sliced

- 2 tablespoons olive oil

- Salt and pepper to taste

- 4 large whole wheat or spinach tortillas

- 1 cup hummus

- Handful of baby spinach leaves

- Crumbled feta cheese for garnish (optional)

Instructions:

1. Preheat the oven to 400°F (200°C).

2. Place sliced vegetables on a baking sheet lined with parchment paper. Drizzle with olive oil and season with salt and pepper. Toss to coat evenly.

3. Roast vegetables in the preheated oven for 20-25 minutes, or until tender and caramelized, stirring halfway through.

4. Warm tortillas in a dry skillet or microwave for a few seconds to make them pliable.

5. Spread a generous layer of hummus onto each tortilla.

6. Top the hummus with roasted vegetables and a handful of baby spinach leaves.

7. Optional: Sprinkle crumbled feta cheese over the vegetables.

8. Roll up the tortillas tightly, tucking in the sides as you go, to form wraps.

9. Slice the wraps in half diagonally before serving, if desired.

10. Serve immediately as a delicious and satisfying lunch or dinner option.

52. Berry and Spinach Salad with Balsamic Vinaigrette

Ingredients:

- 4 cups baby spinach leaves

- 1 cup mixed berries (such as strawberries, blueberries, and raspberries)

- 1/4 cup chopped pecans or walnuts, toasted

- 1/4 cup crumbled goat cheese or feta cheese

- 2 tablespoons balsamic vinegar

- 1 tablespoon extra virgin olive oil

- 1 teaspoon honey

- Salt and pepper to taste

Instructions:

1. In a large bowl, combine baby spinach leaves, mixed berries, chopped toasted nuts, and crumbled goat cheese or feta cheese.

2. In a small bowl, whisk together balsamic vinegar, extra virgin olive oil, honey, salt, and pepper to make the vinaigrette.

3. Drizzle the balsamic vinaigrette over the salad and toss until everything is well coated.

4. Serve immediately as a refreshing and nutritious salad.

53.Lemon Herb Baked Salmon

Ingredients:

- 4 salmon fillets

- Salt and pepper to taste

- Zest and juice of 1 lemon

- 2 tablespoons olive oil

- 2 cloves garlic, minced

- 1 teaspoon dried thyme

- 1 teaspoon dried rosemary

- Fresh parsley for garnish (optional)

Instructions:

1. Preheat the oven to 375°F (190°C). Line a baking sheet with parchment paper.

2. Season salmon fillets with salt and pepper on both sides.

3. In a small bowl, whisk together lemon zest, lemon juice, olive oil, minced garlic, dried thyme, and dried rosemary.

4. Place salmon fillets on the prepared baking sheet. Pour the lemon herb mixture over the salmon, ensuring it is evenly coated.

5. Bake in the preheated oven for 12-15 minutes, or until salmon is cooked through and flakes easily with a fork.

6. Remove from the oven and garnish with fresh parsley before serving.

54. Quinoa Stuffed Bell Peppers

Ingredients:

- 4 large bell peppers, halved and seeds removed
- 1 cup quinoa, rinsed
- 2 cups vegetable broth or water
- 1 tablespoon olive oil
- 1 onion, diced
- 2 cloves garlic, minced
- 1 zucchini, diced
- 1 carrot, diced
- 1 cup diced tomatoes
- 1 teaspoon dried oregano
- 1 teaspoon dried basil
- Salt and pepper to taste

- 1/2 cup shredded mozzarella cheese

- Fresh basil leaves for garnish (optional)

Instructions:

1. Preheat the oven to 375°F (190°C). Lightly grease a baking dish.

2. In a saucepan, combine quinoa and vegetable broth or water. Bring to a boil, then reduce heat to low, cover, and simmer for 15-20 minutes, or until quinoa is cooked and liquid is absorbed. Remove from heat and let it cool slightly.

3. In a skillet, heat olive oil over medium heat. Add diced onion and minced garlic. Sauté until onions are translucent and fragrant.

4. Add diced zucchini and diced carrot to the skillet. Cook until vegetables are softened.

5. Stir in diced tomatoes, dried oregano, dried basil, salt, and pepper. Cook for another 2-3 minutes to combine flavors.

6. In a large bowl, combine cooked quinoa with the vegetable mixture.

7. Arrange bell pepper halves in the prepared baking dish. Spoon the quinoa and vegetable mixture into each pepper half.

8. Sprinkle shredded mozzarella cheese over the stuffed peppers.

9. Cover the baking dish with aluminum foil and bake in the preheated oven for 25-30 minutes, or until peppers are tender and cheese is melted.

10. Garnish with fresh basil leaves before serving.

55.Caprese Pasta Salad

Ingredients:

- 8 ounces pasta (such as fusilli or penne)

- 1 cup cherry tomatoes, halved

- 1 ball fresh mozzarella cheese, diced

- 1/4 cup chopped fresh basil leaves

- 2 tablespoons extra virgin olive oil

- 1 tablespoon balsamic vinegar

- Salt and pepper to taste

- Grated Parmesan cheese for garnish (optional)

Instructions:

1. Cook pasta according to package instructions until al dente. Drain and rinse under cold water to cool.

2. In a large bowl, combine cooked pasta, cherry tomatoes, diced mozzarella cheese, and chopped fresh basil.

3. Drizzle extra virgin olive oil and balsamic vinegar over the pasta salad. Toss until everything is well coated.

4. Season with salt and pepper to taste.

5. Serve chilled or at room temperature, optionally garnished with grated Parmesan cheese.

56.Black Bean and Corn Salad

Ingredients:

- 1 can (15 ounces) black beans, drained and rinsed

- 1 cup corn kernels (fresh, frozen, or canned)

- 1 bell pepper, diced

- 1/4 cup red onion, finely chopped

- 1/4 cup chopped fresh cilantro

- Juice of 1 lime

- 2 tablespoons extra virgin olive oil

- 1 teaspoon ground cumin

- Salt and pepper to taste

- Avocado slices for garnish (optional)

- Tortilla chips for serving (optional)

Instructions:

1. In a large bowl, combine black beans, corn kernels, diced bell pepper, chopped red onion, and chopped fresh cilantro.

2. In a small bowl, whisk together lime juice, extra virgin olive oil, ground cumin, salt, and pepper to make the dressing.

3. Pour the dressing over the black bean and corn mixture. Toss until everything is well coated.

4. Taste and adjust seasoning if needed.

5. Garnish with avocado slices before serving, if desired.

6. Serve chilled as a refreshing and flavorful salad, accompanied by tortilla chips if desired.

57.Ratatouille

Ingredients:

- 1 eggplant, diced

- 2 zucchini, diced

- 1 bell pepper, diced

- 1 onion, diced

- 2 cloves garlic, minced

- 2 tomatoes, diced

- 2 tablespoons tomato paste

- 1 teaspoon dried thyme

- 1 teaspoon dried oregano

- Salt and pepper to taste

- Fresh basil leaves for garnish (optional)

Instructions:

1. Heat some olive oil in a large skillet or Dutch oven over medium heat.

2. Add diced eggplant to the skillet and cook until softened and slightly browned. Remove from the skillet and set aside.

3. In the same skillet, add more olive oil if needed, then add diced zucchini and cook until slightly softened. Remove from the skillet and set aside.

4. Add diced bell pepper and diced onion to the skillet. Cook until onions are translucent and peppers are softened.

5. Stir in minced garlic and cook until fragrant, about 1 minute.

6. Return cooked eggplant and zucchini to the skillet. Add diced tomatoes, tomato paste, dried thyme, dried oregano, salt, and pepper. Stir to combine.

7. Cover the skillet and let the ratatouille simmer over low heat for 20-25 minutes, stirring occasionally, until vegetables are tender and flavors are well blended.

8. Taste and adjust seasoning if needed.

9. Garnish with fresh basil leaves before serving.

58.Mediterranean Chickpea Salad

Ingredients:

- 2 cans (15 ounces each) chickpeas, drained and rinsed

- 1 cucumber, diced

- 1 bell pepper, diced

- 1/4 cup red onion, finely chopped

- 1/4 cup Kalamata olives, pitted and chopped

- 1/4 cup crumbled feta cheese

- 2 tablespoons chopped fresh parsley

- 2 tablespoons extra virgin olive oil

- 2 tablespoons lemon juice

- 1 teaspoon dried oregano

- Salt and pepper to taste

Instructions:

1. In a large bowl, combine chickpeas, diced cucumber, diced bell pepper, chopped red onion, chopped Kalamata olives, crumbled feta cheese, and chopped fresh parsley.

2. In a small bowl, whisk together extra virgin olive oil, lemon juice, dried oregano, salt, and pepper to make the dressing.

3. Pour the dressing over the chickpea salad. Toss until everything is well coated.

4. Taste and adjust seasoning if needed.

5. Serve chilled or at room temperature as a flavorful and satisfying salad.

59. Spinach and Mushroom Quiche

Ingredients:

- 1 pre-made pie crust (store-bought or homemade)

- 1 tablespoon olive oil

- 8 ounces mushrooms, sliced

- 2 cups fresh spinach leaves

- 1/2 cup diced onion

- 4 large eggs

- 1 cup milk or half-and-half

- 1 cup shredded Swiss cheese

- Salt and pepper to taste

- Pinch of nutmeg (optional)

- Fresh parsley for garnish (optional)

Instructions:

1. Preheat the oven to 375°F (190°C). Place the pie crust in a pie dish and crimp the edges.

2. In a skillet, heat olive oil over medium heat. Add sliced mushrooms and diced onion. Cook until mushrooms are golden brown and onions are translucent.

3. Add fresh spinach leaves to the skillet and cook until wilted. Remove from heat and let it cool slightly.

4. In a mixing bowl, whisk together eggs and milk (or half-and-half). Season with salt, pepper, and a pinch of nutmeg if using.

5. Spread the mushroom, spinach, and onion mixture evenly over the bottom of the pie crust. Sprinkle shredded Swiss cheese over the top.

6. Pour the egg mixture over the filling in the pie crust.

7. Bake in the preheated oven for 35-40 minutes, or until the quiche is set and the crust is golden brown.

8. Remove from the oven and let it cool for a few minutes before slicing.

9. Garnish with fresh parsley before serving.

60.Greek Orzo Salad

Ingredients:

- 1 cup orzo pasta

- 2 cups cherry tomatoes, halved

- 1 cucumber, diced

- 1/4 cup red onion, finely chopped

- 1/4 cup Kalamata olives, pitted and chopped

- 1/4 cup crumbled feta cheese

- 2 tablespoons chopped fresh parsley

- 2 tablespoons extra virgin olive oil

- 2 tablespoons lemon juice

- 1 teaspoon dried oregano

- Salt and pepper to taste

Instructions:

1. Cook orzo pasta according to package instructions until al dente. Drain and rinse under cold water to cool.

2. In a large bowl, combine cooked orzo pasta, cherry tomatoes, diced cucumber, chopped red onion, chopped Kalamata olives, crumbled feta cheese, and chopped fresh parsley.

3. In a small bowl, whisk together extra virgin olive oil, lemon juice, dried oregano, salt, and pepper to make the dressing.

4. Pour the dressing over the orzo salad. Toss until everything is well coated.

5. Taste and adjust seasoning if needed.

6. Serve chilled or at room temperature as a refreshing and flavorful salad.

61.Baked Sweet Potato Fries

Ingredients:

- 2 large sweet potatoes, peeled and cut into fries

- 2 tablespoons olive oil

- 1 teaspoon paprika

- 1/2 teaspoon garlic powder

- 1/2 teaspoon onion powder

- Salt and pepper to taste

- Chopped fresh parsley for garnish (optional)

Instructions:

1. Preheat the oven to 425°F (220°C). Line a baking sheet with parchment paper.

2. In a large bowl, toss sweet potato fries with olive oil, paprika, garlic powder, onion powder, salt, and pepper until evenly coated.

3. Spread the seasoned sweet potato fries in a single layer on the prepared baking sheet.

4. Bake in the preheated oven for 20-25 minutes, flipping halfway through, until fries are crispy and golden brown.

5. Garnish with chopped fresh parsley before serving.

62.Lemon Garlic Roasted Broccoli

Ingredients:

- 1 large head of broccoli, cut into florets

- 2 tablespoons olive oil

- 3 cloves garlic, minced

- Zest and juice of 1 lemon

- Salt and pepper to taste

- Grated Parmesan cheese for garnish (optional)

Instructions:

1. Preheat the oven to 425°F (220°C). Line a baking sheet with parchment paper.

2. In a large bowl, toss broccoli florets with olive oil, minced garlic, lemon zest, lemon juice, salt, and pepper until evenly coated.

3. Spread the seasoned broccoli florets in a single layer on the prepared baking sheet.

4. Roast in the preheated oven for 20-25 minutes, or until broccoli is tender and lightly browned, stirring halfway through.

5. Sprinkle with grated Parmesan cheese before serving, if desired.

63.Lentil and Vegetable Soup

Ingredients:

- 1 cup dried lentils

- 4 cups vegetable broth

- 1 onion, diced

- 2 carrots, diced

- 2 stalks celery, diced

- 2 cloves garlic, minced

- 1 can (14 ounces) diced tomatoes

- 1 teaspoon dried thyme

- 1 teaspoon dried rosemary

- Salt and pepper to taste

- Chopped fresh parsley for garnish (optional)

Instructions:

1. In a large pot, combine dried lentils and vegetable broth. Bring to a boil, then reduce heat to low, cover, and simmer for 20-25 minutes, or until lentils are tender.

2. In a separate skillet, heat some olive oil over medium heat. Add diced onion, diced carrots, diced celery, and minced garlic. Sauté until vegetables are softened.

3. Add sautéed vegetables to the pot with cooked lentils and vegetable broth.

4. Stir in diced tomatoes, dried thyme, dried rosemary, salt, and pepper.

5. Let the soup simmer for an additional 10-15 minutes to allow flavors to meld together.

6. Taste and adjust seasoning if needed.

7. Garnish with chopped fresh parsley before serving.

64.Grilled Vegetable Skewers

Ingredients:

- Assorted vegetables (such as bell peppers, zucchini, mushrooms, cherry tomatoes, and red onion), cut into chunks

- 2 tablespoons olive oil

- 2 cloves garlic, minced

- 1 teaspoon dried oregano

- 1 teaspoon dried basil

- Salt and pepper to taste

- Wooden skewers, soaked in water for 30 minutes

Instructions:

1. Preheat the grill to medium-high heat.

2. In a large bowl, toss vegetable chunks with olive oil, minced garlic, dried oregano, dried basil, salt, and pepper until evenly coated.

3. Thread the seasoned vegetable chunks onto the wooden skewers, alternating different vegetables.

4. Grill the vegetable skewers for 10-12 minutes, turning occasionally, until vegetables are tender and lightly charred.

5. Remove from the grill and serve hot as a delicious and nutritious side dish or appetizer.

65.Quinoa Stuffed Acorn Squash

Ingredients:

- 2 acorn squash, halved and seeds removed

- 1 cup quinoa, rinsed

- 2 cups vegetable broth or water

- 1 tablespoon olive oil

- 1 onion, diced

- 2 cloves garlic, minced

- 1 carrot, diced

- 1 celery stalk, diced

- 1/4 cup dried cranberries or raisins

- 1/4 cup chopped pecans or walnuts

- 1 teaspoon dried thyme

- Salt and pepper to taste

- Fresh parsley for garnish (optional)

Instructions:

1. Preheat the oven to 400°F (200°C). Place the acorn squash halves, cut side down, on a baking sheet lined with parchment paper. Bake for 25-30 minutes, or until squash is tender when pierced with a fork.

2. In a saucepan, combine quinoa and vegetable broth or water. Bring to a boil, then reduce heat to low, cover, and simmer for 15-20 minutes, or until quinoa is cooked and liquid is absorbed. Remove from heat and let it cool slightly.

3. In a skillet, heat olive oil over medium heat. Add diced onion and minced garlic. Sauté until onions are translucent and fragrant.

4. Add diced carrot and diced celery to the skillet. Cook until vegetables are softened.

5. Stir in dried cranberries or raisins, chopped pecans or walnuts, dried thyme, cooked quinoa, salt, and pepper. Cook for another 2-3 minutes to combine flavors.

6. Spoon the quinoa mixture into the roasted acorn squash halves.

7. Return stuffed squash to the oven and bake for an additional 10-15 minutes, or until heated through.

8. Garnish with fresh parsley before serving.

66.Greek Lemon Chicken Soup (Avgolemono)

Ingredients:

- 6 cups chicken broth
- 1/2 cup uncooked orzo pasta
- 3 eggs
- Juice of 2 lemons
- 2 cups shredded cooked chicken
- Salt and pepper to taste
- Chopped fresh dill for garnish (optional)

Instructions:

1. In a large pot, bring chicken broth to a boil. Add uncooked orzo pasta and cook until al dente, according to package instructions.

2. In a mixing bowl, whisk together eggs and lemon juice until well combined.

3. Gradually whisk in a ladleful of hot chicken broth into the egg-lemon mixture, stirring constantly.

4. Slowly pour the egg-lemon mixture back into the pot with the remaining chicken broth and orzo pasta, stirring constantly.

5. Add shredded cooked chicken to the soup. Season with salt and pepper to taste.

6. Let the soup simmer for a few minutes until heated through.

7. Taste and adjust seasoning if needed.

8. Serve hot, garnished with chopped fresh dill if desired.

67.Roasted Beet and Goat Cheese Salad

Ingredients:

- 4 medium beets, peeled and cut into wedges

- 2 tablespoons olive oil

- Salt and pepper to taste

- 4 cups mixed salad greens

- 1/2 cup crumbled goat cheese

- 1/4 cup chopped walnuts or pecans, toasted

- Balsamic vinaigrette dressing

Instructions:

1. Preheat the oven to 400°F (200°C). Line a baking sheet with parchment paper.

2. Toss beet wedges with olive oil, salt, and pepper until evenly coated. Spread them in a single layer on the prepared baking sheet.

3. Roast in the preheated oven for 30-35 minutes, or until beets are tender and caramelized, stirring halfway through.

4. In a large bowl, combine mixed salad greens with roasted beet wedges, crumbled goat cheese, and toasted nuts.

5. Drizzle with balsamic vinaigrette dressing and toss until everything is well coated.

6. Serve immediately as a delicious and colorful salad option.

68.Teriyaki Tofu Stir-Fry

Ingredients:

- 14 ounces extra firm tofu, pressed and cubed

- 2 tablespoons soy sauce

- 2 tablespoons honey or maple syrup

- 1 tablespoon rice vinegar

- 1 teaspoon sesame oil

- 2 cloves garlic, minced

- 1 teaspoon grated ginger

- 1 tablespoon cornstarch

- 2 tablespoons water

- 2 tablespoons vegetable oil

- 1 bell pepper, sliced

- 1 cup broccoli florets

- 1 carrot, sliced

- Cooked rice for serving

- Sesame seeds for garnish (optional)

- Sliced green onions for garnish (optional)

Instructions:

1. In a small bowl, whisk together soy sauce, honey or maple syrup, rice vinegar, sesame oil, minced garlic, and grated ginger to make the teriyaki sauce.

2. In another small bowl, mix cornstarch and water to make a slurry.

3. Heat vegetable oil in a large skillet or wok over medium-high heat.

4. Add cubed tofu to the skillet and cook until golden brown on all sides. Remove tofu from the skillet and set aside.

5. In the same skillet, add sliced bell pepper, broccoli florets, and sliced carrot. Stir-fry until vegetables are tender-crisp.

6. Return cooked tofu to the skillet. Pour the teriyaki sauce over the tofu and vegetables.

7. Stir in the cornstarch slurry to thicken the sauce.

8. Cook for another 1-2 minutes, stirring constantly, until the sauce is thickened and everything is well coated.

9. Serve hot over cooked rice, garnished with sesame seeds and sliced green onions if desired.

69.Coconut Curry Lentil Soup

Ingredients:

- 1 tablespoon coconut oil
- 1 onion, diced
- 2 cloves garlic, minced
- 1 tablespoon grated ginger
- 2 tablespoons curry powder
- 1 cup dried red lentils
- 4 cups vegetable broth
- 1 can (14 ounces) coconut milk
- 2 cups spinach leaves
- Juice of 1 lime
- Salt and pepper to taste
- Chopped fresh cilantro for garnish (optional)
- Cooked rice for serving

Instructions:

1. In a large pot, heat coconut oil over medium heat. Add diced onion, minced garlic, and grated ginger. Sauté until onions are translucent and fragrant.

2. Stir in curry powder and cook for another minute to toast the spices.

3. Add dried red lentils and vegetable broth to the pot. Bring to a boil, then reduce heat to low, cover, and simmer for 15-20 minutes, or until lentils are cooked and tender.

4. Stir in coconut milk and spinach leaves. Cook for another 5 minutes, until spinach is wilted and flavors are well combined.

5. Remove from heat and stir in lime juice. Season with salt and pepper to taste.

6. Serve hot over cooked rice, garnished with chopped fresh cilantro if desired.

70. Berry Chia Seed Pudding

Ingredients:

- 1/4 cup chia seeds

- 1 cup almond milk or coconut milk

- 1 tablespoon honey or maple syrup

- 1/2 teaspoon vanilla extract

- Mixed berries for topping (such as strawberries, blueberries, and raspberries)

- Granola for topping (optional)

Instructions:

1. In a bowl, whisk together chia seeds, almond milk or coconut milk, honey or maple syrup, and vanilla extract.

2. Cover and refrigerate for at least 2 hours or overnight, until the chia seeds have absorbed the liquid and the mixture has thickened to a pudding-like consistency.

3. Stir the chia pudding well before serving.

4. Divide the pudding into serving bowls and top with mixed berries and granola, if desired.

5. Serve chilled as a delicious and nutritious dessert or breakfast option.

71.Mediterranean Chickpea and Quinoa Salad

Ingredients:

- 1 cup quinoa, rinsed
- 2 cups water or vegetable broth
- 1 can (15 ounces) chickpeas, drained and rinsed
- 1 cucumber, diced
- 1 bell pepper, diced
- 1/4 cup red onion, finely chopped
- 1/4 cup Kalamata olives, pitted and chopped
- 1/4 cup crumbled feta cheese
- 2 tablespoons chopped fresh parsley
- 2 tablespoons extra virgin olive oil
- 2 tablespoons lemon juice
- 1 teaspoon dried oregano
- Salt and pepper to taste

Instructions:

1. In a saucepan, combine quinoa and water or vegetable broth. Bring to a boil, then reduce heat to low, cover, and simmer for 15-20 minutes, or until quinoa is cooked and liquid is absorbed. Remove from heat and let it cool slightly.

2. In a large bowl, combine cooked quinoa, chickpeas, diced cucumber, diced bell pepper, chopped red onion, chopped Kalamata olives, crumbled feta cheese, and chopped fresh parsley.

3. In a small bowl, whisk together extra virgin olive oil, lemon juice, dried oregano, salt, and pepper to make the dressing.

4. Pour the dressing over the salad. Toss until everything is well coated.

5. Taste and adjust seasoning if needed.

6. Serve chilled or at room temperature as a flavorful and satisfying salad.

72.Roasted Garlic and Cauliflower Soup

Ingredients:

- 1 head cauliflower, cut into florets

- 2 tablespoons olive oil

- Salt and pepper to taste

- 1 head garlic

- 2 tablespoons butter or olive oil

- 1 onion, diced

- 4 cups vegetable broth

- 1/2 cup heavy cream or coconut milk (for a dairy-free option)

- Chopped fresh chives for garnish (optional)

- Croutons for garnish (optional)

Instructions:

1. Preheat the oven to 400°F (200°C). Line a baking sheet with parchment paper.

2. Place cauliflower florets on the prepared baking sheet. Drizzle with olive oil and season with salt and pepper. Toss to coat evenly.

3. Cut the top off the head of garlic to expose the cloves. Drizzle with olive oil, wrap in aluminum foil, and place on the baking sheet with the cauliflower.

4. Roast in the preheated oven for 25-30 minutes, or until cauliflower is tender and lightly browned, and garlic cloves are soft and caramelized.

5. In a large pot, melt butter or heat olive oil over medium heat. Add diced onion and cook until translucent.

6. Squeeze the roasted garlic cloves out of their skins and add them to the pot with the onions.

7. Add roasted cauliflower florets to the pot and pour in vegetable broth. Bring to a simmer and cook for 15-20 minutes.

8. Use an immersion blender or transfer the soup to a blender to puree until smooth.

9. Stir in heavy cream or coconut milk to the desired consistency.

10. Season with salt and pepper to taste.

11. Serve hot, garnished with chopped fresh chives and croutons if desired.

73.Turkey and Vegetable Skillet

Ingredients:

- 1 tablespoon olive oil

- 1 pound ground turkey

- 1 onion, diced

- 2 cloves garlic, minced

- 1 bell pepper, diced

- 1 zucchini, diced

- 1 cup cherry tomatoes, halved

- 1 teaspoon dried oregano

- 1 teaspoon dried basil

- Salt and pepper to taste

- Cooked quinoa or rice for serving

- Fresh parsley for garnish (optional)

Instructions:

1. Heat olive oil in a large skillet over medium heat. Add ground turkey and cook until browned, breaking it up with a spoon.

2. Add diced onion and minced garlic to the skillet. Cook until onions are translucent and fragrant.

3. Stir in diced bell pepper, diced zucchini, cherry tomatoes, dried oregano, dried basil, salt, and pepper. Cook for another 5-7 minutes, or until vegetables are tender.

4. Serve hot over cooked quinoa or rice, garnished with fresh parsley if desired.

74.Sweet and Spicy Glazed Salmon

Ingredients:

- 4 salmon fillets
- Salt and pepper to taste
- 2 tablespoons honey
- 2 tablespoons soy sauce
- 1 tablespoon sriracha sauce (adjust to taste)
- 1 tablespoon rice vinegar
- 1 teaspoon minced ginger
- 2 cloves garlic, minced
- Sesame seeds for garnish (optional)
- Sliced green onions for garnish (optional)

Instructions:

1. Preheat the oven to 400°F (200°C). Line a baking sheet with parchment paper.

2. Season salmon fillets with salt and pepper on both sides, then place them on the prepared baking sheet.

3. In a small bowl, whisk together honey, soy sauce, sriracha sauce, rice vinegar, minced ginger, and minced garlic to make the glaze.

4. Brush the glaze over the salmon fillets, ensuring they are evenly coated.

5. Bake in the preheated oven for 12-15 minutes, or until salmon is cooked through and flakes easily with a fork.

6. Remove from the oven and garnish with sesame seeds and sliced green onions before serving.

75.Ratatouille Stuffed Bell Peppers

Ingredients:

- 4 bell peppers, halved and seeds removed

- 1 eggplant, diced

- 2 zucchini, diced

- 1 onion, diced

- 2 cloves garlic, minced

- 2 tomatoes, diced

- 2 tablespoons tomato paste

- 1 teaspoon dried thyme

- 1 teaspoon dried oregano

- Salt and pepper to taste

- Olive oil for cooking

- Fresh basil leaves for garnish (optional)

Instructions:

1. Preheat the oven to 375°F (190°C). Lightly grease a baking dish.

2. Heat olive oil in a large skillet over medium heat. Add diced onion and minced garlic. Sauté until onions are translucent and fragrant.

3. Add diced eggplant and diced zucchini to the skillet. Cook until vegetables are softened.

4. Stir in diced tomatoes, tomato paste, dried thyme, dried oregano, salt, and pepper. Cook for another 2-3 minutes to combine flavors.

5. Arrange bell pepper halves in the prepared baking dish. Spoon the ratatouille mixture into each pepper half.

6. Cover the baking dish with aluminum foil and bake in the preheated oven for 25-30 minutes, or until peppers are tender.

7. Remove from the oven and garnish with fresh basil leaves before serving.

76.Avocado Tuna Salad

Ingredients:

- 2 cans (5 ounces each) tuna, drained

- 2 ripe avocados, diced

- 1/4 cup diced red onion

- 1/4 cup diced celery

- 1/4 cup chopped fresh cilantro

- Juice of 1 lime

- Salt and pepper to taste

- Whole grain bread or lettuce leaves for serving

Instructions:

1. In a large bowl, combine drained tuna, diced avocado, diced red onion, diced celery, chopped fresh cilantro, and lime juice.

2. Gently toss until ingredients are well combined.

3. Season with salt and pepper to taste.

4. Serve the avocado tuna salad on whole grain bread as sandwiches or wrapped in lettuce leaves for a low-carb option.

77.Mediterranean Grilled Chicken Kabobs

Ingredients:

- 1 pound boneless, skinless chicken breasts, cut into chunks
- 1 bell pepper, cut into chunks
- 1 red onion, cut into chunks
- 1 zucchini, sliced
- 1/4 cup olive oil
- 2 tablespoons lemon juice
- 2 cloves garlic, minced
- 1 teaspoon dried oregano
- 1 teaspoon dried basil
- Salt and pepper to taste
- Wooden skewers, soaked in water for 30 minutes

Instructions:

1. In a bowl, whisk together olive oil, lemon juice, minced garlic, dried oregano, dried basil, salt, and pepper to make the marinade.

2. Place the chicken chunks in the marinade, coating them evenly. Cover and refrigerate for at least 30 minutes, or overnight for best results.

3. Preheat the grill to medium-high heat.

4. Thread marinated chicken chunks onto skewers, alternating with bell pepper, red onion, and zucchini slices.

5. Grill the kabobs for 10-12 minutes, turning occasionally, until chicken is cooked through and vegetables are tender.

6. Serve hot as a delicious and protein-packed meal.

78.Roasted Brussels Sprouts with Balsamic Glaze

Ingredients:

- 1 pound Brussels sprouts, trimmed and halved

- 2 tablespoons olive oil

- Salt and pepper to taste

- 2 tablespoons balsamic vinegar

- 1 tablespoon honey or maple syrup

- 1 teaspoon Dijon mustard

- 1 garlic clove, minced

- Chopped fresh parsley for garnish (optional)

Instructions:

1. Preheat the oven to 400°F (200°C). Line a baking sheet with parchment paper.

2. In a bowl, toss Brussels sprouts with olive oil, salt, and pepper until evenly coated.

3. Spread Brussels sprouts in a single layer on the prepared baking sheet.

4. Roast in the preheated oven for 20-25 minutes, or until Brussels sprouts are golden brown and tender, stirring halfway through.

5. In a small saucepan, combine balsamic vinegar, honey or maple syrup, Dijon mustard, and minced garlic. Bring to a simmer over medium heat and cook for 2-3 minutes, stirring constantly, until the glaze thickens slightly.

6. Drizzle the roasted Brussels sprouts with the balsamic glaze.

7. Garnish with chopped fresh parsley before serving.

79. Berry Spinach Salad with Poppy Seed Dressing

Ingredients:

- 4 cups baby spinach leaves

- 1 cup mixed berries (such as strawberries, blueberries, and raspberries)

- 1/4 cup sliced almonds, toasted

- 2 tablespoons crumbled feta cheese

- 2 tablespoons olive oil

- 1 tablespoon apple cider vinegar

- 1 tablespoon honey

- 1 teaspoon Dijon mustard

- 1 teaspoon poppy seeds

- Salt and pepper to taste

Instructions:

1. In a large bowl, combine baby spinach leaves, mixed berries, toasted sliced almonds, and crumbled feta cheese.

2. In a small bowl, whisk together olive oil, apple cider vinegar, honey, Dijon mustard, poppy seeds, salt, and pepper to make the dressing.

3. Drizzle the dressing over the salad and toss until everything is well coated.

4. Serve immediately as a refreshing and nutritious salad option.

80. Lemon Herb Grilled Shrimp

Ingredients:

- 1 pound large shrimp, peeled and deveined

- 2 tablespoons olive oil

- Zest and juice of 1 lemon

- 2 cloves garlic, minced

- 1 tablespoon chopped fresh parsley

- 1 teaspoon dried oregano

- Salt and pepper to taste

- Wooden skewers, soaked in water for 30 minutes

Instructions:

1. In a bowl, whisk together olive oil, lemon zest, lemon juice, minced garlic, chopped fresh parsley, dried oregano, salt, and pepper to make the marinade.

2. Add the peeled and deveined shrimp to the marinade, tossing to coat evenly. Cover and refrigerate for 30 minutes.

3. Preheat the grill to medium-high heat.

4. Thread marinated shrimp onto skewers.

5. Grill the shrimp skewers for 2-3 minutes per side, or until shrimp are pink and opaque.

6. Serve hot as a flavorful and protein-rich dish.

81.Quinoa and Black Bean Stuffed Peppers

Ingredients:

- 4 bell peppers, halved and seeds removed

- 1 cup quinoa, rinsed

- 2 cups vegetable broth

- 1 can (15 ounces) black beans, drained and rinsed

- 1 cup corn kernels

- 1/2 cup diced tomatoes

- 1/2 cup shredded cheese (such as cheddar or pepper jack)

- 1 teaspoon chili powder

- 1/2 teaspoon cumin

- Salt and pepper to taste

- Chopped fresh cilantro for garnish (optional)

Instructions:

1. Preheat the oven to 375°F (190°C). Lightly grease a baking dish.

2. In a saucepan, combine quinoa and vegetable broth. Bring to a boil, then reduce heat to low, cover, and simmer for 15-20 minutes, or until quinoa is cooked and liquid is absorbed. Remove from heat and let it cool slightly.

3. In a large bowl, combine cooked quinoa, black beans, corn kernels, diced tomatoes, shredded cheese, chili powder, cumin, salt, and pepper.

4. Arrange bell pepper halves in the prepared baking dish. Spoon the quinoa and black bean mixture into each pepper half.

5. Cover the baking dish with aluminum foil and bake in the preheated oven for 25-30 minutes, or until peppers are tender.

6. Remove from the oven and garnish with chopped fresh cilantro before serving.

== THE END ==

Thank you for choosing our book! We trust that it met or exceeded your expectations.

If you enjoyed our book, kindly consider sharing your thoughts in a review on social media. Your feedback is invaluable as it aids us in enhancing our products and services for future readers.

We sincerely appreciate your support and extend our best wishes to you.